LEMON ESSENTIAL OIL

Manage Your Weight And Transform Your Health With The Power Of Lemon Essential Oils And Bioactive Food

Markus Helen

Table of Contents

CHAPTER ONE

INTRODUCTION TO LEMON ESSENTIAL OIL

Lemon critical oil is a very herbal factor that still serves as a domestic fitness remedy. It's extracted from the peel of fresh lemons the use of a "cold-pressing" manner that pricks and rotates the peel as oil is released.

Lemon critical oil may be diluted and carried out topically on your pores and skin, as nicely as subtle into the air and inhaled. Some humans swear via way of means of lemon critical oil as an factor that fights exhaustion, facilitates with despair, clears your pores and skin, kills dangerous viruses and micro organism, and decreases inflammation.

In latest years, the scientific literature has commenced to seize up with the claims made via way of means of humans who've used lemon critical oil for years. Read directly to research extra approximately the advantages of lemon critical oil, viable aspect results of the use of it, and extra.

May lessen tension and despair signs and symptoms

You may also have observed that after you operate lemon-scented merchandise for cleansing your domestic, you experience extra comfortable and in a higher temper afterward.

Of course, a number of that is probably the herbal end result of sharpening up your environment; however the real heady fragrance of lemons in all likelihood performs a element in that calming feeling.

A Source done on mice confirmed that lemon critical oil become a effective calming and temper-enhancing agent all through 3 pressure check experiments.

The identical examine concluded that lemon critical oil become extra powerful at relieving pressure than different critical oils together with lavender and rose.

There are promising signs that diffusing lemon essential oil has an impact on assuaging a few signs and symptoms of tension and despair.

ILLNESS SIGNS AND SYMPTOMS

Nausea and vomiting are of the maximum not unusual place signs and symptoms skilled in early pregnancy.

There can be motive to trust that lemon critical oil can relieve (or as a minimum lower) the severity of those signs and symptoms.

In a Source of a hundred pregnant girls, aromatherapy with lemon critical oil become located to lower the stages of nausea and vomiting significantly.

Can make your pores and skin healthier.

CHAPTER TWO

BENEFITS OF ESSENTIAL OIL

Lemon oil is one in every of numerous critical oils which could kill dangerous micro organism which could develop for your pores and skin.

In a latest Source, lemon critical oil becomes proven to be powerful in opposition to lines of micro organism like Staphylococcus aurous and E. coli. This makes an excellent desire for topically cleansing small wounds.

Other studies has showed lemon critical oil's impact in opposition to contamination inflicting micro organism and can save you pores and skin inflammation, such as a laboratory examine carried out.

It additionally has protecting residences, together with antioxidants, which could brighten and maintain your pores and skin tone.

CAN ACT AS A ACHE RELIEVER

Lemon essential oil is every now and then utilized in aromatherapy as a herbal analgesic. The anti-pressure and antidepressant results of this oil may also have something to do with the way it facilitates our bodies interpret our ache without panicking.

Lemon oil aromatherapy modified the manner the animals' brains spoke back to painful stimuli.

To decide how lemon oil impacts people who're in ache, extra studies is needed. May assist you breathe less difficult and soothe a sore throat If you've got a chilly or are experiencing a sore throat, lemon critical oil is an excellent domestic remedy to try.

Try putting in a diffuser with lemon oil to launch its sweet, tangy heady fragrance for your room even as you get a few rest. The calming residences of lemon oil can assist loosen up each your thoughts and the muscle mass for your throat.

There isn't a variety of medical information that backs up lemon oil aromatherapy with calming the not cold, however we do understand that the nutrition C and antioxidant residences of lemon juice are of advantage while you simply want to respire a bit less difficult.

It's viable that the residences of lemon critical oil paintings in tons the identical manner while you deal with a sore throat with aromatherapy.

Remember, it's now no longer secure to ingest critical oils.

Helps you experience alert and focused

Lemon critical oil perks up your temper; however it additionally may go to reinforce your brainpower.

May be powerful in treating and stopping zits breakouts

When diluted and carried out topically, lemon critical oil can kill micro organism which could get trapped in pores and purpose breakouts. It also can make clear your pores and skin with antioxidants and nutrition C, lightly exfoliating lifeless pores and skin cells that so frequently come to be trapped in hair follicle and pores.

Since lemon oil has recovery residences, you get the delivered bonus of quicker recovery from breakouts and remedy of your zits scars while you operate it.

May sell wound recovery

Since lemon critical oil is full of nutrition C, antioxidants, and antimicrobial residences, it won't wonder you to research that this oil may belong for your first useful resource kit. lemon critical oil promoted quicker recovery of tissue inflamed with mange.

You can cleanse the region of a small reduce or scrape with diluted lemon oil to sanitize it, discourage contamination, and in all likelihood assist the wound heal extra quickly.

Have antifungal residences.

CHAPTER THREE

BENEFIT OF LEMMON ESSENTIAL OIL

Lemon critical oil has effective antifungal residences for treating sure pores and skin overgrowths. In fact, a overview of Source notes it's powerful in opposition to fungi that purpose athlete's foot, thrush, and yeast infections while carried out topically.

POTENTIAL ASPECT RESULTS

Like the alternative critical oils within side the citrus family, lemon critical oil is commonly secure for topical and aromatherapy use. Notably, it's pronounced to be secure for pregnant girls and toddlers over 3 months old.

There are case Source of lemon critical oil making your pores and skin extra touchy to inflammation from the solar so it's miles nice to keep away from direct daylight while the use of any citrus critical oil.

This inflammation is referred to as photo toxicity, and it reasons a brief redness that appears much like slight sunburn. You may additionally experience a uncooked or burning sensation for your pores and skin within side the region in which you've carried out lemon oil.

You can typically keep away from hypersensitivity via way of means of well diluting any critical oil you operate and doing a patch check for your pores and skin earlier than you try and use it on a bigger region.

Lemon oil isn't permitted as secure to be used on animals. Some critical oils could have a poisonous impact while ingested or inhaled via way of means of pets. Think approximately your hairy pals that are probably close by while you inhale aromatherapy.

HOW TO APPLY THIS ESSENTIAL OIL

You can adequately use lemon critical oil via way of means of diffusing it or making use of it topically.

To diffuse lemon critical oil, area 3 or 4 drops within side the diffuser of your desire. Make positive you're in a nicely-ventilated region, and restrict your aromatherapy classes to 30 minutes.

To use lemon critical oil topically, blend it nicely with a provider oil of your desire.

Test the combination on a small, inconspicuous region of your pores and skin earlier than you practice it someplace touchy, like your face. If after 24 hours you notice redness or inflammation, don't use the combination.

To keep away from pores and skin damage, make certain you wash off lemon oil earlier than exposing your pores and skin to daylight.

WHY ARE LEMON ESSENTIAL OIL OILS IMPORTANT?

Topical lemon critical oil is secure to use immediately for your pores and skin — if you operate a provider oil. Carrier oils are noncorrosive, less-focused oils that won't damage the outer layer of your pores and skin.

To dilute critical oils adequately, upload approximately 12 drops of your critical oil to each ounce of your base, or provider oil. Popular provider oils include almond oil, jojoba oil, and coconut oil.

Essential oils aren't meals-grade merchandise and aren't examined via way of means of the Food and Drug Administration (FDA) for safety. Lemon critical oils incorporate risky elements, which imply they could oxidize and sooner or later cross bad.

Purchasing an lemon oil may be a chunk tricky. There are masses of manufacturers that promote mixed critical oil merchandise that declare to be beneficial, however those merchandise have numerous substances except oils.

Look for oil this is cold-pressed and a hundred percentage pure. Check the substances listing earlier than you're making an critical oil purchase.

Purchase lemon critical oil at your nearby fitness meals save or store online.

The takeaway

Lemon essential oil is an anti inflammatory and antimicrobial factor that will let you enhance your temper, locate intellectual clarity, lessen pressure, and extra.

Remember, simply due to the fact a product is deemed "herbal" doesn't imply that it doesn't deliver viable aspect results. Never practice lemon oil immediately on your pores and skin with out a provider oil, and in no way ingest any critical oil.

Essential oils aren't a substitute for prescription remedies out of your doctor, however they could paintings as a awesome supplement on your ordinary fitness and health routine.

THE END

www.ingramcontent.com/pod-product-compliance
Lightning Source LLC
Chambersburg PA
CBHW071020260726
48662CB00022B/961